HOMEMADE BEAUTY PRODUCTS

The Definitive Guide To Looking Naturally Beautiful

KATE ANDERSON

© 2015

Copyright © 2015 by Kate Anderson
Publishing

"A girl should be two things: who and what she wants."

Coco Chanel

Table Of Contents

Looking Naturally Beautiful

In this day and age, there is an astounding amount of pressure to look our best. The world around us is intensely focused on looking younger, healthier, and blemish free. We are all influenced by things like the media, celebrity magazines and websites that focus heavily on our looks. Advertisements for creams, gadgets, cosmetic procedures and surgeries are everywhere. As time goes on, it is impossible to ignore that there is more and more importance placed on how we appear to others. We may feel like we are being compared to other people in our age bracket. We may feel pressured to look our best when we are competing for a certain job or position in our current careers. With so much focus being placed on our looks, it's hard not to get swept away in the ever growing tide of the cosmetic industry.

On average, American women spend $160,000 on beauty products and procedures in their lifetime and this is only increasing. Cosmetic surgical and nonsurgical procedures such as Botox and liposuction have gone up 446% in the last 10 years. Today, little girls are getting manicures and pedicures before they even reach double digits. They are also getting not only their legs waxed, but even their bikini lines! Teenage girls are getting nose jobs and breast augmentations before even reaching university age.

In addition to being swayed by the media and advertising campaigns, women today are working longer hours and being subjected to increasing levels of stress. If we are working long hours we might not be sleeping enough so our eyes may appear puffy and discoloured. If we're overly busy, we may be skipping meals or grabbing faster foods that are not only full of fats, salts, and sugars, but are also lacking essential vitamins and minerals which may hold the key to keeping us naturally beautiful. The more caught up we are with the quickening pace of the world, the pressure to be beautiful is becoming insurmountable, and as the pressure increases, so do the sales of chemical based beauty treatments.

Unfortunately, the problems we are facing as a result of these changing times extend far beyond our pocketbooks. Our self esteems are lowered, our body image is becoming warped, and a whole new generation of "mean girls" is rising like a phoenix (albeit a very well made-up, cellulite-free phoenix). And what's worse is that most of us have no idea what is actually IN our beauty products. Nor are we schooled on the damage it's actually causing to our health and our environment!

The fact is, most of us are consumed with our looks even if we don't want to be. And the pressure is there whether we like it or not. It's in our careers, it's at the school yard, it's in our own homes! This book is not going to tell you to stop caring about your looks! The intention here is to open your mind to the possibility of alternative ways of caring for your skin rather than relying on chemical based cosmetics. This way you will not only save yourself thousands of dollars in your lifetime, you will also protect yourself and our environment from the effects of harmful chemicals.

This book will discuss what's really in your favourite products, how to avoid harmful chemicals, and how to take better care of your body naturally. In addition, I will supply you with numerous recipes for homemade body scrubs and other organic cosmetic products that will leave your skin looking and feeling luscious without any detrimental effects to your health OR your pocketbook!

What's Really In Your Beauty Products. The Shocking Truth.

Surveys have shown that the average woman uses around 13 products a day. It has been estimated that women use around 515 chemicals on their skin before they even leave the house in the morning! Nowadays, we are smothering ourselves in countless chemicals that may have detrimental effects on our health and our environment. Most of our beauty products contain at least 20 ingredients; many of which may be doing more harm than good.

Have a look at the list of ingredients on any single product on your vanity table right now and see if you know what any of them actually are? Chances are, you don't, and if you don't know what it is, it's safe to assume that you don't know where it comes from, nor what harm it could potentially have on your health. Nor will you know what effect it has on the environment and wildlife once it gets washed down your drain. Most of our favourite cosmetic products are packed with industrially produced, dangerous chemicals. And guess what! They are not only harmful to your health and the environment. Some studies have shown that your "anti-ageing" regime may actually be causing you to age even faster.

We all have favourite products. Whether it's our face masks, our cellulite scrubs, or even our dental hygiene products, we love our products for the results they have on our looks. We can see the effects of some beauty products instantly which might give an instant boost to our confidence; however, this could also mean that we end up believing that chemical based treatments are the only way to achieve these results and that's just not true.

Most of us would like to believe that our favourite products wouldn't be on the market if they weren't safe to use so we brush off any concern about those long lists of ingredients. Rather than worrying about what these chemicals actually are we focus instead on what we expect them to do. We put our trust in the belief that our governments would protect us from harmful chemicals by not allowing them to remain on the market. Unfortunately, the world doesn't work that way.

The laws regulating the use of most of the harmful chemicals in beauty products are loose at best. Firstly, the cumulative effects of these products is a very valid concern that simply cannot be answered with the type of basic study that goes into deeming products "safe" for use. The fact is, most of us use multiple products at once and it is simply impossible to know which products are being used in conjunction with others. Just because a product is deemed to be harmless or "safe" does not mean it is harmless when used with other products.

If a certain chemical is deemed to be safe at certain levels, what happens if you are using multiple products containing the same ingredient at the same time? You could easily be slathering your skin in toxic levels of chemicals without even realising it. Think of pharmaceutical drugs. Your doctor or pharmacist will always flag up drug interactions to ensure your safety. Unfortunately, the same procedure is not taken for things like beauty products. Furthermore, few of us even consider what sort of effects our products could have on us if used over an extensive period of time. There is little research showing the effects of long term use of beauty products. So, whereas your doctor will tell you when to discontinue using a medication that isn't suitable for long term use, your beautician is highly unlikely to follow suit.

One in eight of the 82,000 ingredients commonly used in beauty products are industrial chemicals; many of which are also used in products such as household cleaners, automotive degreasers, surfactants (used in things like paint and ink), and plasticisers (used in concrete). These chemicals have been proven to be responsible for numerous health problems; the least of which are allergies and skin sensitivities; the more serious of which are fertility and reproductive problems, hormonal disturbances, and a variety of cancers. As you can imagine these chemicals aren't exactly environmentally friendly nor can they validate any claims of being "kind" to your skin.

Below is a list of the most harmful offenders that may be lurking on your vanity table. Check all your cosmetics, hair care, and dental care products for these chemicals. If you discover any product listing these harmful chemicals consider getting rid of them, replacing them, or at least reducing your use of them. Consider extending your search to any products your children use and your household cleaners.

The 12 Chemicals In Beauty Products You MUST Avoid!

1. BHA (butylated hydroxyanisole) and BHT (butylated hydroxytoluene)

Used mainly in moisturisers and makeup as preservatives. Research of both BHA and BHT have produced significantly varied findings, offering results ranging from harmless to highly toxic. The fact that results vary so much could lead to further concern regarding the unpredictability of these chemicals in humans. Some reports have found these preservatives to be suspected endocrine disruptors and carcinogens (BHA). They have been proven to be harmful to fish and other wildlife.

2. Coal tar dyes: p-phenylenediamine and colours listed as "CI" followed by a five digit number *(U.S. colour name may also be listed e.g. "FD&C Blue No. 1" or "Blue 1")*

Coal tar dyes are artificial colouring agents. They are made by combining hydrocarbons like toluene, xylene, benzene, which are obtained from the distillation of bituminous coal. Coal tars are also made from petroleum distillates. These colouring agents are used in cosmetics, hair dyes, deodorants, and shampoos. Studies have shown that coal tar dyes can cause skin reactions and allergies. That have also been linked to ADHD, hyperactivity, and learning difficulties in children. Other studies have implicated a connection between coal tar dyes and skin and lung cancers, though a direct link has not been proven as of yet.

3. DEA (Diethanolamine)

Used as a wetting agent in creamy and foaming products, such as shampoos, lotions and other cosmetics. DEA itself is not harmful; however, it can react with other ingredients in cosmetic products to form a very potent carcinogen called nitrosodiethanolamine (NDEA) which is easily absorbed through the skin. It has been linked with cancers of the stomach, liver, oesophagus, and bladder. DEA and NDEA are also harmful to fish and other wildlife.

DEA related ingredients may be listed in a variety of ways including:
* Cocamide DEA
* Cocamide MEA
* DEA-Cetyl Phosphate
* DEA Oleth-3 Phosphate
* Lauramide DEA
* Linoleamide MEA
* Myristamide DEA
* Oleamide DEA
* Stearamide MEA
* TEA-Lauryl Sulfate
* Triethanolamine

4. Dibutyl phthalate (DBP)

Used in nail care products and other cosmetics. DBP is readily absorbed through the skin. It has been shown to cause developmental defects, reduced sperm counts, and changed in the testes and prostate. DBP is also a suspected endocrine disrupter on the grounds that evidence shows that it interferes with hormone function and it may cause harm to an unborn child. DBP is also harmful to fish and other wildlife. It is often used in fragrances so avoid it by using products that are "fragrance free" or "unscented".

5. Formaldehyde-releasing preservatives

Formaldehyde-releasing preservatives are added to products to keep them from growing bacteria and increase their shelf life. They can be absorbed through the skin and may cause irritation to skin and eyes, and trigger allergies. These preservatives slowly release formaldehyde (a known human carcinogen) which may cause serious health risks when inhaled. It is also possibly persistent in the environment.

Formaldehyde-releasing preservatives may be listed as:
* DMDM hydantoin
* diazolidinyl urea
* imidazolidinyl urea
* methenamine
* quarternium-15
* sodium hydroxymethylglycinate

6. Parabens

Used in a variety of cosmetics such as shampoos, hair gels, body lotions, and shaving gels as preservatives. The use of parabens is becoming increasingly controversial as studies are showing direct links between them and a some serious health problems including fertility issues in men and breast cancer. Despite claims made by cosmetic companies stating that parabens can't be absorbed into skin, research shows that anywhere between 20 and 60 per cent of them can be absorbed into the body.

7. Parfum (a.k.a. fragrance)

All cosmetics that contain any fragrances will have the word 'parfum' on the ingredients list. It is important to note that products labelled as "fragrance-free" or "unscented" may include any mixture of fragrance ingredients to cover any chemical scent that may be in a product. Some fragrance ingredients can trigger allergies and asthma while others are linked to cancer and neurotoxicity. Some are harmful to fish and other wildlife.

8. Polyethylene glycols (PEG compounds)

PEGs are petroleum-based compounds that are widely used in cosmetic cream bases. PEGs may be contaminated with measurable amounts of ethylene oxide and 1,4-dioxane, both of which are potential human carcinogens. While carcinogenic contaminants are the primary concern, PEG compounds themselves show some evidence of genotoxicity. If used on broken skin they may cause irritation and even systemic toxicity. Look for related chemical propylene glycol and other ingredients with the letters "eth" (e.g., polyethylene glycol).

9. Petrolatum

Found in lip balms, hair care products, soaps, and other cosmetics. Petrolatum is used in hair products to add shine to your hair and also acts as a moisture barrier (i.e. in lip balms or lipsticks). This chemical can be contaminated with polycyclic aromatic hydrocarbons, which may cause cancer. Petrolatum is considered a carcinogen and is restricted for use in cosmetics in the European Union.

10. Siloxanes

Siloxanes, derived from silicone, are widely used in the cosmetics industry. They add beneficial qualities such as spreadability, enhanced skin feel, reduction in greasiness, increased absorption, amongst other benefits we look for in our cosmetic products. Unfortunately, though siloxanes may work wonders on your skin and hair, they are packed with health risks. They are known endocrine disruptors, are proven to interfere with hormone function and potentially impair fertility. Research has shown that siloxanes can cause uterine tumours and derail the functioning of neurotransmitters in the nervous system. These also pose serious harm to the environment, aquatic life, and wild life. Look for ingredients ending in "-siloxane" or "-methicone."

Look out for these alternate listing names:
cyclotetrasiloxane
cylcopentasiloxane
cyclohexasiloxane
cyclomethicone

11. Sodium Laureth Sulfate (SLES) or Sodium Lauryl Sulfate (SLS)

Used in foaming cosmetics, such as shampoos, toothpastes, mouthwashes, soaps, bubble baths, body washes, and more. SLS is used widely due to its effectiveness as a cleaner and its inexpensive cost. SLS is under considerable debate regarding its safety. There are many claims linking SLS with cancer however those claims are as yet unproven. Studies have shown side effects such as skin irritation and skin corrosion at very low levels of concentration. It has also been found to have residual levels in the liver, lungs, brain, and heart and studies have indicated that SLS will remain in a person's system for up to 5 days.

Research has shown links to hormone levels with symptoms ranging from PMS to menopause. A lower rate of male fertility has also been reported, as has poor eye development in children. One serious concern is that SLS can become contaminated with 1,4-dioxane, a suspected carcinogen.

12. Triclosan

Triclosan is an antibacterial and antifungal agent found in cosmetic products such as soaps, toothpastes, and antiperspirants. This chemical has been linked to liver tumours and liver cancers in laboratory mice. Studies suggest the chemical could have similar effects on humans. Triclosan is also a suspected endocrine disrupter and may contribute to antibiotic resistance in bacteria. What is most shocking is that, though Triclosan is a synthetic compound not found in nature, it has been reportedly found in the breast milk 97 per cent of lactating women. This chemical is also harmful to fish and other wildlife.

"It's nice to just embrace the natural beauty within you."
Victoria Justice

Part Two: The Better Ways!

Most women absolutely love their products. We talk about them with our friends and family. We read reviews about them online and in magazines. We search for products that will magically produce the results we desire; a younger looking face, the cure for our unwanted lumps and bumps, hair that isn't frizzy, too straight, or too curly. We love our products because they work well (most of the time). We're always excited to try a new product. And most importantly, we love them because we feel like we're treating ourselves every time we use them. We feel a lift to our self esteem. We feel luxurious.

If you feel reluctant to give up your beauty products, don't worry. You don't have to give everything up to make a difference to your health and live a more environmentally friendly life. There are plenty of simple things you can do to right now to make a change. The following list shows some simple ways you can change your habits to limit the harm done to yourself and the world around you without getting rid of all your favourite products.

16 Easy Ways To Make A Change IMMEDIATELY!

1 - Use fewer products!
Have a look at your skin regime and see where you may be using two or more products for the same thing. Cut down to one product wherever possible.

2 - Use less of everything.
When it comes to things like shampoo, make-up, body lotion, and toothpaste, most of us use far more than is actually necessary. Instead of slathering your skin in large quantities of creams or make-up products, use a smaller amount. Use only as much as you really NEED.

3 - Take a day off.
If you wear make up on a daily basis, try to cut out at least one day a week to let your skin breathe. Doing this means that not only are you sparing yourself the chemicals for a day, you are also ensuring a healthier complexion which means you'll need less products in the future!

4 - Let your skin breathe!
If you suffer from acne breakouts, rather than using extra make up to cover them up, let your skin breathe as often as possible by avoiding make-up whenever possible. Combat your breakouts by avoiding excess sugar in your diet, keeping hair off your face, touching your face less, and washing your face regularly (at least morning and night and after any exercise, sun exposure, or swimming).

5 – Keep your products clean!
Wash your facecloths and replace heads on facial brushes regularly. Bacteria and fungi can grow on wash cloths that are left dirty or wet and these could cause break outs, irritation, or infection.

6 – Avoid!
Avoid harmful hair treatments such as perms, colourings, and excess washing.

7 – Dry Hair
If your hair is dry or frizzy, rather than using products to "tame" it, try leaving a day or two between washes to allow the natural oils in your scalp to nourish your hair. When you wash your hair, remember to use the shampoo on your scalp and the conditioner on your hair.

8 – Water. And lots of it!
Drink at least 8 glasses of water per day to keep your skin youthful, supple, and blemish free.

9 – Foods to avoid

Avoid foods high in fats, salt, and sugar. Steer clear of processed foods, junk food, and take away foods.

10 – Sleep!

Be sure to get your beauty rest! Being tired can make you look washed out or puffy which may mean you're wearing more make-up than you need to. Get regular, good quality sleep to avoid looking run down.

11 - Stop smoking!

We all know that cigarette smoke can cause very serious illness. It can also cause unsightly discolouration to your teeth, bad breath, and signs of premature ageing such as lines, wrinkles, thin lips, and eye bags. Avoid smoking and you will need less products to make you look healthy.

12 - Stay out of the sun!

Too much exposure to the sun can be detrimental to your health. It can also leave your skin dry and discoloured which may mean you are using more products to combat and cover up its effects than necessary.

13 – Drinks to avoid.

Avoid drinking too much alcohol and caffeine to keep from becoming dehydrated.

14 - Get regular exercise.

Exercise plays an important role in our overall health and mental wellbeing. If you're having difficulties sleeping or managing your stress levels, it will show on your skin. Exercising regularly is a great natural way to stay healthy and calm which keep your face looking naturally great.

15 - Stress management.
If your face is showing signs of stress you may feel the need to use more make-up or chemical treatments. Practice relaxation, make time for socialising and recreation, and get plenty of fresh air.

16 - Be a pro-active consumer.
If you don't want to make your own products at home, choose safer, more natural store-bought products. Be sure to check the ingredients so you can be certain of a product's safety.

In the next part of this book I'm going to show you how you can nourish your body from within and turn your favourite "superfoods" into homemade cleansers and body scrubs, but before we get to the fun stuff, how about a little eye opener?

Remember that up to 60% of chemicals used in your daily beauty regime can be absorbed through your skin causing detrimental effects to your health. It may be hard to believe that certain chemicals are more likely to enter your bloodstream by being absorbed through your skin than they are through your digestive tract; however, it's the truth.

In addition to discussing the potential danger of certain chemicals, earlier in this text I discussed how your favourite anti-ageing products may actually be making you age faster. In the list that follows I will show you some common products that may be doing more harm than good. I will also include some very common bad habits that you may want to avoid.

"You really don't need to wear any make-up most of the time; keep your eyebrows the way they are, and find your own natural beauty signature."
Erin Heatherton

10 Common Habits and Products To Avoid

1 - Permanent and Semi-permanent Hair Dyes

Studies have linked long term hair dye use to bladder confer, multiple myeloma, and non-Hodgkin's lymphoma.

2 - Compound Henna Hair Dye

Any henna hair dye includes metallic salts for pigmentation despite being advertised as being "all natural" and often without it even being mentioned on the label. If you're not scared away by future health problems, think about this: if you've used a compound henna hair product you MUST wait at least a year or two before using any chemical hair dye containing hydrogen peroxide. If you don't, you risk ending up with greenish-black hair and you may end up with a rather unpleasant odour and smoke being emitted from your head. This might be okay for Halloween, but might not be great for the office.

3 - Sleeping with your hair out

This isn't going to cause you serious bodily harm but if you suffer from acne or if you want to cut down on the amount of products you use in general, tie your hair back at night and be sure you clip your bangs away from your face. Your hair contains oils which can cause oily complexion and may cause breakouts.

4 - Picking at your face

Whether you're popping pimples or just generally over-grooming, picking at your face will not only leave you with scars and wrinkles, it will also leave your pores and sores wide open and ready to absorb whatever product or make-up product you put on next which could cause irritation and faster absorption of toxic chemicals into your blood stream.

5 - Exfoliating too much or too often

Exfoliating should take no longer than one minute and should be done a maximum of two to three times a week. When you over-exfoliate, you are removing a protective layer of skin leaving your skin exposed to sun damage and chemical damage you may accrue from subsequent product or make-up use. This ultimately leaves your skin prone to signs of ageing thereby negating any positive effect you may have desired from exfoliating in the first place.

6 - Eye Shadows and Eyeliner With Aluminium Powder

Darker or brighter coloured eye shadows and eyeliners that contain aluminium powder have been linked to neurotoxicity and cancer. Beware: This ingredient is not only found in cheaper products so don't be fooled into thinking you're safe by choosing a product with a larger number on the price tag.

7 - Mineral Make-up

Make-ups that advertise "natural" mineral ingredients could be causing you more harm than chemical based powders and lipsticks. Minerals such as iron oxides are often found in association with toxic metals such as mercury and lead. Although these are often only found in small quantities, this is a good example of a product that can build up in the body over time. It can therefore be a serious risk for health problems in the future. For happier pores and ultimate safety, wear less make-up less often or avoid wearing it all together.

8 - Using dirty make-up brushes

I spoke earlier about the importance of cleaning and replacing your face cloths and cleansing brushes, the same applies to your make-up brushes. Your foundation brush specifically is clinging on to daily dirt and bacteria. Invest in a brush cleaner and replace all make-up tools regularly to avoid irritation and infection.

9 – Antiperspirants

The use of aluminium salts in antiperspirants has been linked to breast cancer, reproductive failure, and ovarian lesions. In addition to the damage being done by aluminium, most antiperspirants also feature paragons and phthalates. To keep yourself safe, try a natural deodorant. Some of these work better than others so be sure to try more than one before giving up. Also, don't forget that adding ANY product to skin that has just been shaven will increase the rate of chemicals being absorbed into your bloodstream and can also cause local skin irritation. Always wait an hour or more after shaving your underarms before applying your antiperspirant.

10 – Perfumes

Notoriously full of secret ingredients, the use of perfumes is linked to allergic reaction and hormone disruption. The worst thing about perfume reactions is they often come from someone else wearing the perfume nearby (similar to second-hand smoking). Allergic reactions to perfumes aren't always just mild bouts of sneezing, they can also trigger asthma attacks, nausea, and migraines.

Part 3: Take easy action TODAY!

Now that you know what not to do, it's time to start looking at what you should do to keep your skin, hair, and nails healthy and beautiful the natural way. I often wonder why it is that most of us believe in brand names and new chemical formulas more than we believe in natural sources of vitamins and minerals that have been proven to be good for us for centuries. We all know how important it is to eat well for good health. If someone put a table full of fresh ingredients in front of you beside a frozen microwavable dinner and asked you which one was healthier, I doubt anyone would have any difficulty answering correctly!

We think about taking care of our organs in a ton of ways. We don't smoke for the sake of our lungs, we don't drink too much to keep our liver healthy, we eat healthier foods for our stomachs, blood pressure, and cholesterol. But for some reason, we often forget that our skin is an organ too and it needs the same nourishment as the rest of our body. And the same goes for your hair, nail, and teeth.

What you put in your body is just as, if not more important than what you put on it. Imagine lining your stomach or lungs with your favourite shampoo or skin cream. You'd never do that, because you know it's poison right? So why is it we don't think twice about slathering these things on our skin?

Impurities that show on our skin, eyes, teeth, and hair are often a result of an unhealthy diet or lifestyle. Therefore it is extremely important to treat your body kindly in order to keep you looking younger and healthier. There are many foods that contain vital nutrients for the health of your skin, hair, teeth and nails. These foods are not only good for your looks, they'll also keep you feeling great too!

Remember that in order keep your body at optimum levels of health, you should keep your diet varied. Offer your body a variety of sources of proteins, vitamins, fatty acids, and minerals rather than relying on one or two sources on repeat. A varied diet will not only keep your body happier, it will also keep you from falling into boring cycles of eating the same old foods every day! Nourish your skin from the inside out by including the following "superfoods" into your diet.

16 Superfoods For Your Skin, Hair, And Nails

1 – Blueberries
Packed with Anthocyanins, blueberries are a powerful antioxidant. Eating a small handful every day will defend you against free radicals that may cause wrinkles and sagging skin.

2 - Wild Salmon
A great source of omega-3 fatty acids, wild salmon (as opposed to farm-raised salmon) can fight inflammation and keep your skin naturally moisturised from the inside out. This means a reduction in acne, eczema, psoriasis, and rosacea as well as overall younger looking skin. Wild salmon is also a great source of selenium which can help protect skin from sun exposure and it contains vitamin D which is beneficial to your teeth, bones, and even your mood!

3 – Spinach
Like most dark leafy greens, there is no end to the benefits of spinach. A great source of vitamins B,C, and E, calcium, iron, magnesium, omega-3 fatty acids, and potassium. Spinach also contains Lutein which keeps your eyes healthy and clear.

4 - Sweet Potatoes
Not only are sweet potatoes delicious and a much healthier spud to have on your plate, they also contain beta-carotene which can help brighten up dull-looking skin, battle fine lines and wrinkles, and fight acne.

5 - Green Beans

This summer vegetable is fantastic for your hair and nails. If you'd like longer, thicker hair and stronger nails, take advantage of the silicon naturally occurring in green beans to treat yourself from the inside out.

6 – Oysters

This fantastic source of zinc will help renew and repair skin cells and keep your hair, nails, and eyes healthy. They may also have a good effect on your love life!

7 – Tomatoes

Packed with powerful anti-ageing antioxidant lycopene, tomatoes are fantastic for keeping your skin looking and feeling great. And the best thing is that - unlike most fruits and vegetables - tomatoes actually function better when they've been cooked or processed. This means that you can feel good about using canned tomatoes, ketchup, and drinking an occasional Bloody Mary!

8 - Walnuts

Another great source of omega-3 fatty acids and vitamin E, just a few of these a day could mean brighter eyes, stronger bones, healthier hair, and smoother skin.

9 - Pumpkin seeds

Essential to body function and beauty, a handful of pumpkin seeds per day can help speed up wound healing, build elastic tissue, ensure less wrinkles and acne and provide natural protection against the sun. As an added bonus, pumpkin seeds can also keep your hair healthy and stop it shedding!

10 – Kiwi

This fruit is packed with vitamin C and antioxidants. Its specialty is healthy bones and teeth and keeping your skin wrinkle-free and firm. Kiwis also protect you from heart disease and cancer.

11 - Kale
You may have noticed that kale has become a celebrity vegetable in recent times. That's because it is brimming with vitamin C and what you didn't know, is that vitamin C isn't only good for you when you have colds and flus, it is actually a wizard and keeping skin dryness and wrinkles at bay. In addition to how it improves your looks, kale (along with other dark leafy greens) may even temper the effect of a high-fat diet.

12 - Green Tea
One or two cups a day can counteract the damage of sun, stress, and cigarette smoke on your skin. Green tea has one of the highest concentrations catechins which have anti-inflammatory, antioxidant, and anti-ageing properties. Swapping your coffee with a cup of this magic elixir can prevent tired-looking, dehydrated skin.

13 - Dark Chocolate
Good news everyone! Chocolate with high cocoa content (at least 85%) will keep your skin softer and plumper by improving skin's circulation. Just don't over do it! One ounce (28g) a day is all you need.

14 – Avocados
These guys get a lot of bad press. Yes avocados are "fattening" but it's monounsaturated fat which is actually healthy as it promotes healthy blood flow! This means good things for your complexion and your brain function as well. Not only that, but avocados also have the highest source of vitamin E of any fruit so they will also keep your skin hydrated and maintain skin elasticity.

15 – Beans

A diet full of a variety of beans (red, black, pinto, and kidney) means a high intake of fibre, B-vitamins, potassium, and antioxidants. These are not only great for the digestive tract and brain function, they are also great for your skin cells.

16 - Whole Grains

Switching to brown rice, whole grain breads and pastas, and adding some quinoa, millet and other whole grains to your diet is a great way to boost your intake of vitamin E and zinc which we know are great for the skin. In addition to making us look great, eating whole grains may reduce your risk of heart disease and maintain good brain health. Just remember to add extra cooking time and water to your brown rice!

The Recipes For Looking Naturally Beautiful

When I look at how much time and money we sink into chemical based beauty products, I have to wonder why it is we don't think we'd feel the same excitement when we make something ourselves. Don't you feel proud when you cook something delicious or take some time to bake cakes or cookies instead of buying store bought treats? When you know what's in your food you will naturally feel more confident about its effect on your body. The same goes for beauty products!

Making your own beauty products at home is not nearly as difficult as you may think. It can actually be a lot of fun! This section will offer you a heap of great tips and recipes that will keep you naturally beautiful in safe and effective ways.

Anti-Ageing: Easy Tricks!

Honey
Believe it or not, pure honey is incredible for drawing out skin impurities. It is also a great moisturiser so it really works wonders as an anti-ageing product. Smooth a teaspoon of honey over a freshly cleaned and dried face. Leave for 10 minutes and then rinse.

Orange Juice
As we age, our skin can become a bit dull and drab. Vitamin C is incredible for brightening up dull complexion. In addition, citrus fruits have natural antibacterial properties which will be great for treating skin impurities and removing toxins. Avoid using store bought orange juice as it is likely to be processed. The simplest way is to take a wedge of an orange and squeeze a bit of juice onto a cotton pad. Always treat your face and neck. Use this treatment

regularly for best results. If you have no oranges in the house, try lemon or grapefruit, or if you're feeling really indulgent, use any combination of the three!

White Tea
When brewed with warm water, white tea can greatly reduce puffiness and darkness around your eyes. It's packed with antioxidants so it works as a great treatment for ageing skin. Avoid using hot water as it may reduce the tea's effectiveness. Once you've brewed your tea, soak a face cloth in it, place over your eyes, and relax. You can use this as an all over facial treatment too if you feel your skin needs a little detox. This treatment is also a great way to wind down after a busy day so you'll be feeling a lot of positive effects from this one.

The Wrinkle Killer Recipe

Ingredients
1/4 of an avocado
1 TBSP of honey
3 TBSP of fresh cream

This luscious recipe works miracles on ageing skin. It will ensure good moisture retention and will act as a filler for wrinkles. Combine all the ingredients in a blender until smooth. Apply it to your face and leave for at least one hour. Rinse with warm water and pat dry.

Honey and Egg White Face Mask Recipe

Ingredients
1 TBSP of honey
1 egg white
4 drops of sandalwood essential oil
4 drops of fennel essential oil

Combine ingredients to form a paste. Apply to a clean dry face and neck. Leave for 20 minutes and rinse thoroughly. This recipe will smooth wrinkles, tighten skin, enhance blood circulation, and preserve moisture.

Oatmeal Anti-Ageing Mask Recipe

Ingredients
1/2 cup of butteramilk
2 TBSP of oats
1 TBSP of olive oil
1 teaspoon of almond oil

Warm the oats and buttermilk in a pan until oats are soft. Add the oils, stir and cool. Mix until you have a smooth paste. Apply to a clean face and neck avoiding the delicate skin around your eyes. Leave and relax for 20 - 30 minutes. Rinse thoroughly alternating between warm and cool water.

Dealing With Dry Skin: Easy Tricks!

Olive Oil
The simplest thing you can use to treat your dry skin is pure olive oil. Rub a small amount on your finger tips and gently rub it onto your face and neck before bed. You don't need much, just a drop or two will do. For all over dry skin, add a spoonful of olive oil to your bath, or lightly cover your arms, legs, tummy, and bust after showering. An added bonus to treating your entire body with olive oil is that your skin will be plumper, smoother, and tighter meaning your body will stay looking and feeling young. Remember to keep the temperature of your showers warm rather than hot as your skin will become dryer if subjected to too much hot water.

Milk
For an all over dry skin treatment, add 2 litres of milk to a warm bath, get in and relax. Milk is a natural moisturiser which makes this is a great alternative to scrubs if you have sensitive skin or if you have already used a scrub in the last day or two. Add a couple drops of lavender oil to your bath for extra relaxation.

Sour Cream
Plain sour cream is a great natural moisturiser. Put a few tablespoons of cool sour cream on your face like a mask, leave for 10 minutes and rinse. This is a great way to use up an item in your fridge that might have to be thrown out tomorrow!

Almond Facial Exfoliator Recipe

Ingredients
3 TBSP of fresh cream
1 cup of white sugar
1/2 cup of brown sugar

1/2 cup of ground almonds
2 TBSP of olive oil

This lush facial exfoliator will gently massage away any dull or dead skin cells while adding tons of nutrients and moisture to you face. Combine all ingredients well and store in a securely lidded jar in your refrigerator. Apply to your face and massage in a circular motion for a minute or two. Avoid the skin around your eyes as it is very delicate. Wash the exfoliator off with warm water and follow with a splash of cold water.

Banana Mask Recipe

<u>Ingredients</u>
1 very ripe banana, mashed
1 teaspoon of olive oil
1 TBSP of honey

Mix all ingredients until smooth. Apply to a clean dry face and leave for 10 minutes. Rinse thoroughly. This mask works wonders on dry skin. It is packed with antioxidants and has natural moisturising and soothing effects leaving your skin relaxed and radiant.

Oily or Acne Prone Skin: Easy Tricks

Black Tea
To treat problematic oily skin, soak a face cloth in some warm black tea, lay it over your face, and relax for 10 minutes. Do this whenever you feel your skin could use a reduction in oil levels. If you have chronically oily skin, use this treatment 3 to 5 times per week for longer lasting results.

Egg White
To help draw out impurities and excess oil from your skin, separate the whites from an egg and smooth directly onto your face. Leave for 10 minutes, rinse with warm water, and pat dry. You will feel a tightening effect as the egg whites do their work.

The Instant Spot Remover Recipe

Ingredients
1 teaspoon of Bewer's Yeast
A squeeze of lemon
A drop of water (just enough to form a thick paste)

This little recipe works miracles on blemishes you need to disappear NOW. Combine these ingredients to make a paste. Apply directly to your blemish, cover with a bandage, and leave for 10 minutes. Rinse and pat dry.

The Daily Acne Defender Recipe

<u>Ingredients</u>
3 teaspoons of dried basil
1 cup of boiling water

This toner can be stored in a spray bottle and used daily to keep acne prone skin clear and healthy. The basil in this recipe works as an antibacterial agent so by spritzing this toner on your face or wiping it on with a cotton ball daily, you can ensure your complexion will look clean and feel fresh. Soak the basil leaves in the boiling water, allow to steep and cool. Strain and store in a spray bottle.

All Over Body Care: Easy Tricks For A Beautiful Body Fast!

Coarse Sugar

Don't have enough time to mix up a whole batch of body scrub? Keep a bag of coarse sugar (such as demerara, muscovado, or plain brown sugar) in your bathroom and use it as a quick scrub when you're showering. Sugar scrubs keep your skin tight and free of impurities. If you have 30 extra seconds to spare, add a drop of almond oil or your favourite essential oil to a small handful of sugar, mix it in your hands and then treat your body. This is a great quick treatment if you're planning on going out with bare legs or if you've got little time to prepare for a hot date!

Beer

You may have heard of people using beer as a hair treatment or you may have done this when you were a kid. Beer is a great for adding volume to thin or limp hair. After shampooing, treat your hair with a whole bottle of beer, then rinse. Use beer that is high in yeast content for best results. Avoid using light beer as it won't work nearly as well.

Agave Hand Exfoliator Recipe

Ingredients
1/2 cup of cooked brown rice
1 TBSP of agave nectar
1 TBSP of lemon juice

Get your mitts on this recipe and your tired, dry, or ageing hands will look younger, healthier, and fresher in minutes. Mix all the ingredients well, apply to dry hands and massage into your skin in a circular motion for a minute or two. This recipe is also great for callouses. If you like the results and you have some left over, try giving your feet a nice rub with it too!

Summer Hair Treatment Recipe

Ingredients
1/2 cup of mayonnaise
1 TBSP of coconut oil (may be substituted with olive oil)
1 teaspoon of coconut extract (may be substituted with almond extract)

This 20 minute hair treatment will leave your hair soft, silky, and smooth. Hair that has been chemically treated (or hair that is naturally dry or frizzy) will rejoice after this! Combine all ingredients until they are mixed well, apply to your hair, cover with some plastic kitchen wrap and relax for 20 minutes, then rinse. For especially dry or damaged hair, add a further 10 minutes. Why not try doing one of your facial treatments while your hair is wrapped up for an all over freshen up?

Mint Choc Chip Lip Balm Recipe

Ingredients
1 teaspoon coconut oil
1 teaspoon pure almond oil
1 teaspoon cocoa butter
3-4 drops pure vitamin E oil
1-2 drops pure peppermint extract
3-4 semisweet chocolate chips

This homemade lip balm isn't just safe and effective, it's delicious too! Combine all ingredients in a heat safe bowl. Melt together by placing the bowl over a pot of boiling water being careful not to let the bowl touch the water (the same way you would melt chocolate if you were baking). Stir slowly but continuously until all the ingredients are melted and well combined throughout. Then pour into a small container and allow to cool for an hour. Store this balm in your fridge or handbag. Just be careful not to take it out with you on a hot day as it may melt!

Banoffee Body Scrub Recipe

Ingredients
1 cup of brown sugar
3 very ripe bananas (mashed)

Combine the bananas and sugar until they are well mixed. Don't be afraid to use your hands, just think of it as extra exfoliator for your mitts! Once prepared, use on your entire body for all over exfoliation and added skin tightness or focus on problem areas like the backs of your legs, your tummy, hips, and bum, or your upper arms. Remember when treating your thighs to brush in an upward motion. Massages like this are great for circulation which will keep your skin tight and bright, and they're also great for loosening up cellulite. For added fun, get your partner on board and have a bit of messy playtime!

Sea Salt and Lavender Scrub Recipe

Ingredients
1 cup of sea salt
4 drops of lavender oil
1 TBSP of dried lavender
1 cup of grapeseed oil

Combine salt and dried lavender, add lavender oil and grapeseed oil and mix well. Store this scrub in a lidded jar and use it in the bath or shower whenever you feel like you need an all over body treatment.

The sea salt in this scrub makes it great for dry skin, eczema, acne and other skin impurities. The lavender is great for its calming scent. Note: you can play around with this recipe! If you're not keen on lavender, try a herb or flower that you do like such as rosemary or camomile!

Strawberry Teeth Whitener Recipe

<u>Ingredients</u>
Equal parts of baking soda and pureed strawberries
1 TBSP of olive oil (for after)

I know it seems crazy to imagine that something red could work to whiten your teeth but believe me, it works! Combine the strawberries and baking soda and load up a mouthguard with it. Leave on your teeth for 30 minutes. Finish by swishing olive oil around your mouth for a minute or two and then brush well. Repeat 2 or 3 times per week as needed.

Be beautiful: The easy, fast and safe way!

To conclude, this text shown you that anyone can be naturally beautiful no matter their skin type or budget. In part one I talked extensively about the shocking amount of toxic chemicals found in beauty products that may be doing our bodies and the environment serious harm. For your reference, I included a short, easy to follow list of toxic chemicals that may be in your beauty products. You should refer to this list any time you find yourself questioning the safety of your beauty products. Remember to also look for these chemicals in any other household products.

In part two I showed you a number of ways you can cut down your usage of chemical-based products or cut them out of your regime all together. I also highlighted some common bad habits to avoid and also showed you how even so called "natural" products may be a lot less "safe" than they claim to be. Remember that by even reducing the quantity and amount of products you use, you are making a positive change on your health and the world around you.

In part three I focused on the importance of a good diet and offered you a list of superfoods that will nourish your skin from the inside out. I then showed you how you have, in your kitchen, everything you need to keep your skin looking young, heathy, and vibrant. I offered you a number of easy tips and natural recipes for skin of all types and all over body care. Don't forget that the best way to look your best is to treat yourself from the inside out. Your lifestyle should include a varied diet of good nutrient rich foods, plenty of water, and plenty of rest and relaxation.

My final thought for you is this:
Trust what you know. If you don't know what an ingredient is, don't put it on your skin!